# I Remember Series
# The Seasons

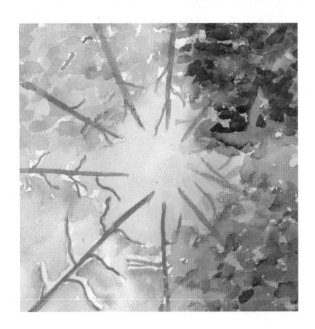

## Brenda C. Poulos
## Illustrated by Janis Cox

Published by Connections Press

Printed in the United States of America

Formatted by Ruth L. Snyder http://ruthlsnyder.com


ISBN: 1544866925

ISBN 13: 978-1544866925


First Edition

To my parents, Ralph and Georgia Schneider. They have been faithful life partners for seventy years.

Dad is now Mom's constant companion and caregiver on her Alzheimer's journey. They are as inseparable as sky and clouds, earth and sea.

# I Remember

My family, my friends,

Things we used to do.

I have memories of my younger days.

I'd like to share with you...

*I Remember the Seasons* is an excellent tool to use with adults diagnosed with Alzheimer's, dementia and other cognitive disorders. It's an amazing conversation starter and reminiscing tool. It can be used to discuss and recall memories from the past.

It's scientifically proven that loved ones who experience Alzheimer's and/or dementia, lose what they learned most recently and keep early childhood memories for the longest.

*I Remember the Seasons* creates endless program opportunities. I recognize this book as one that millions of people and families will cherish. I think it's magnificent work done by Brenda Poulos and Janis Cox. I recommend all long term care facilities and Adult Day programs include this book in their libraries.

I look forward to sharing this book with my clients at the Adult Day program where I work. I know they will enjoy it. It can be utilized in a group setting to run a program or individual Recreation Therapy. This book will enhance families' relationships and communication with their loved ones.

*Georgia Shank, Recreational Therapist*

*"Yet he has not left himself without testimony: He has shown kindness by giving you rain from heaven and crops in their seasons; he provides you with plenty of food and fills your hearts with joy."*

*Acts 14:17*

When my mother was diagnosed with Alzheimer's, I began to research this common form of Dementia. I found that, although short-term memory is commonly lost, millions of people diagnosed with Alzheimer's worldwide still retain many of their childhood memories.

I am convinced that these individuals will be comforted by picture books focusing on many of the things they enjoyed—and still remember—about their early years. Having something in their hands to look at, over and over again, while reliving pleasant times from their past, will serve as a bridge between their present thoughts and memories of days gone by.

When I approached Janis Cox with the idea of a series of picture books for adults with Alzheimer's, it quickly became a collaborative effort that has called both of us to action. It is our hope that our series of Alzheimer's books will be a blessing to yourself and someone you know and love.

*Brenda Poulos*

# The Benefits of Reading Picture Books with People with Alzheimer's

1) Aids in language retention.

2) Helps the brain retain neurological connections.

3) Encourages interactive experiences with the story.

4) Prompts the person to maintain focus and attention.

5) Listening to words and looking at pictures, touching and turning pages, provide a multi-sensory experience.

# How to Use This Book

This book will stimulate the recall of enjoyable memories for people with Alzheimer's, while connecting them in a meaningful way with their caregivers—whether family members or health care professionals. I suggest the following:

- Have the person with Alzheimer's read the text aloud, if he/she would like to and/or is able. If not, it should be read aloud by the caregiver.

- Poems, and illustrations, are followed by *italicized discussion questions*. Please allow time for this activity, for this is key in forming desired connections and developing relationships.

- Utilize the questions as a catalyst for meaningful discussions, rather than accepting answers in a simple "yes" or "no." Talk *with* the person, evoking emotions and helping him/her access past memories as they enjoy forming valuable connections with *you*.

- These questions are merely suggestions. You may substitute, add, or delete them as you see appropriate.

# I Remember the Seasons

Butterflies and flowers,
Camping, swimming, riding bikes.
Roasting marshmallows for hours,
Icicles and snowball fights.

I love the changing seasons.
Summer, autumn, winter, spring.
For each has its own reason
To make my heart sing!

# I Remember
# WINTER

# I Remember
## SLEDDING WITH FRIENDS

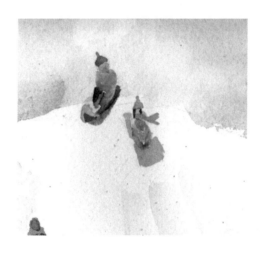

I set my sled on the powdery snow.

We jump aboard and off we go!

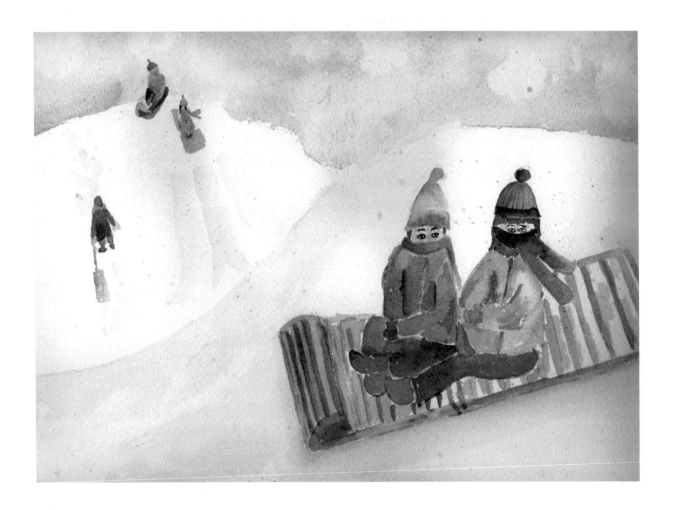

*Who did you go sledding with? What did you like most about your time together? What did you wear to keep you warm while sledding? Did you take a tumble? Tell about it. How did the snow feel? How did it taste?*

# I Remember
## SKATING ON THE POND

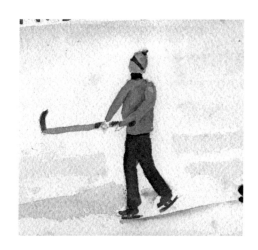

We twirl and glide across the ice.

Skating in winter is mighty nice!

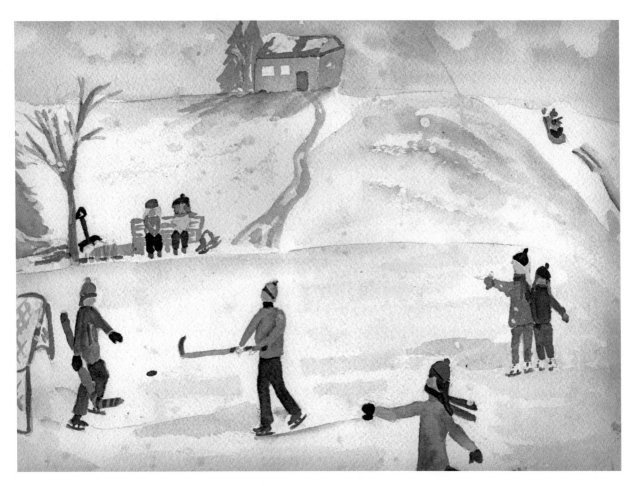

*Did you ice skate on a pond or in an ice skating rink? What games did you play on the ice? Do you remember the wind blowing your hair? What did that feel like? What did twirling on the ice feel like? What did your heart feel like when you skated fast? What caused you to get dizzy? Did you fall? When you fell, how did you feel? Why was it hard to get up again?*

# I Remember
## BUILDING A SNOWMAN

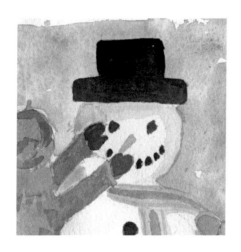

Building a snowman,

Me and my friends.

Laughing and playing,

The fun never ends!

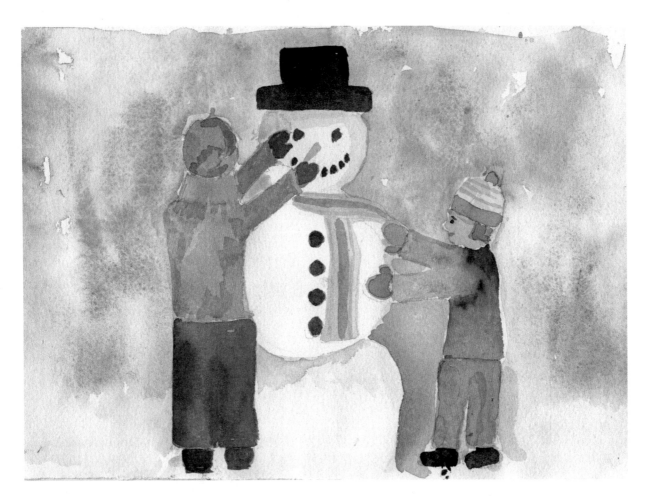

*Who helped you make your snowman? What did you use for his eyes... nose...mouth? How long did he last before he melted? What other activities did you like doing in the snow? What games did you play in the snow?*

# I Remember SPRING

# I Remember
## SPRING FLOWERS

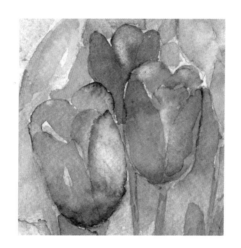

Sun and rain are sure to bring

Lovely flowers that bloom in spring.

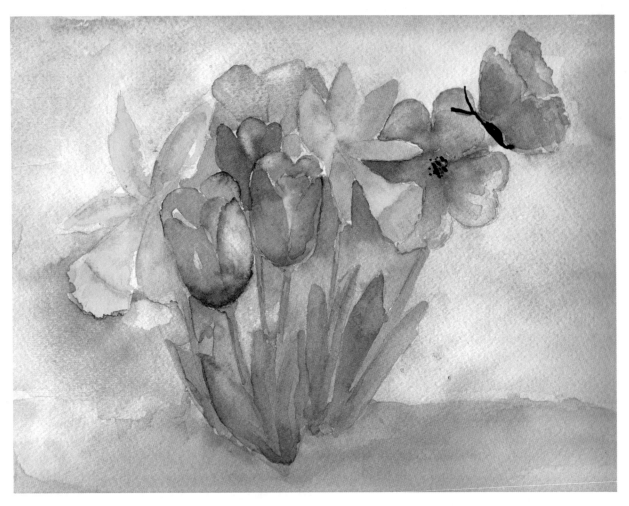

*How do spring flowers smell? Which flowers are your favorites? What colors are they? Have you planted any yourself? Remember the feel of the dirt in your fingers. What was that like? Name the insects that are nearby. If you had a garden, what did you plant in it?*

# I Remember
## FLYING KITES

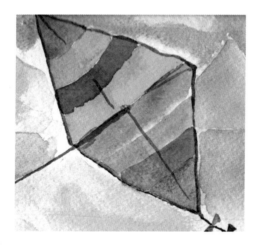

My kite climbs high overhead.

What better reason to get out of bed?

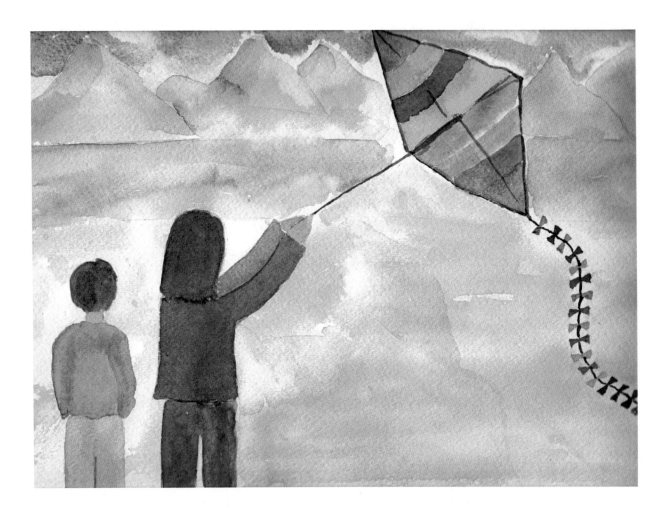

*What did your kite look like? What color was it? What emotions did you feel as it flew in the spring air? Did you have trouble keeping it up in the air on a windy day? Who went kite flying with you?*

# I Remember

## PLAYING BASEBALL

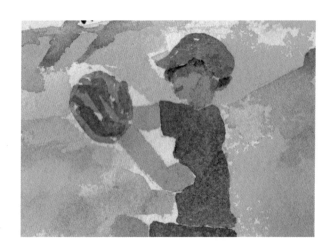

Blue cap, white pants.

Bat held high.

The pitcher winds up.

And lets the ball fly!

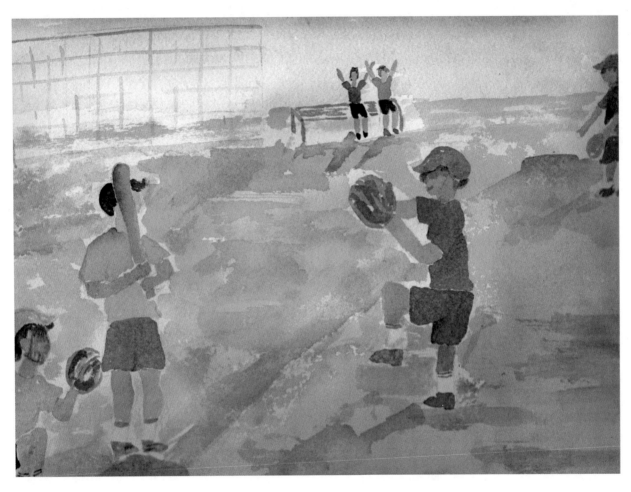

*Did you play baseball or watch as others played? Did you play on a school team or with others in your neighborhood? If you played, how did it feel when you were up to bat? Tell about running the bases. What position did you like to play? What was your team's name?*

# I Remember SUMMER

# I Remember
## RIDING BIKES

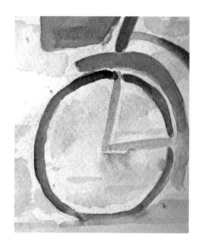

I hop on my bike,

Take off down the street.

Then head for the corner

Where all the kids meet.

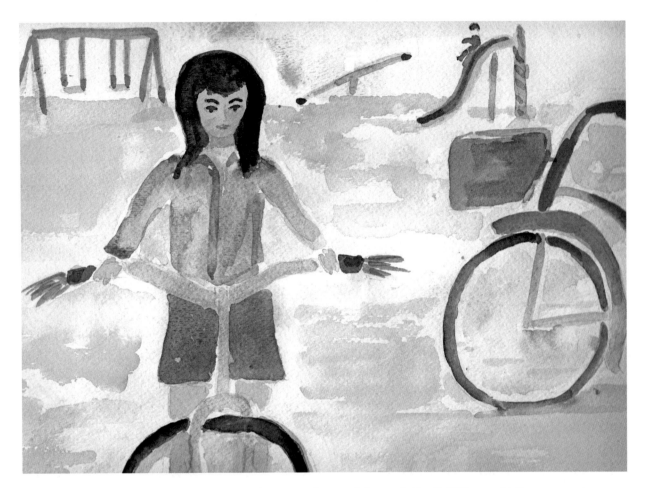

*How old were you when you learned to ride a bike? What did you enjoy most about riding bikes? Who did you ride with? Where did you go? What color was your bicycle? Did it have a bell? What did it sound like? What did you put in the basket? What did it feel like to ride down a hill? Who did you stop to visit or what did you stop to do along the way?*

# I Remember
## CAMPING

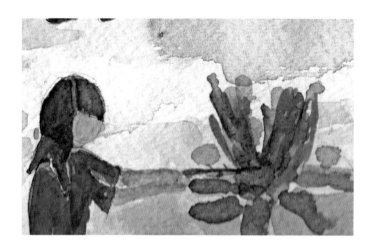

We put up the tent and then went for a hike.

Fished to our heart's content.

Collected rocks and roasted marshmallows.

We're so glad we went!

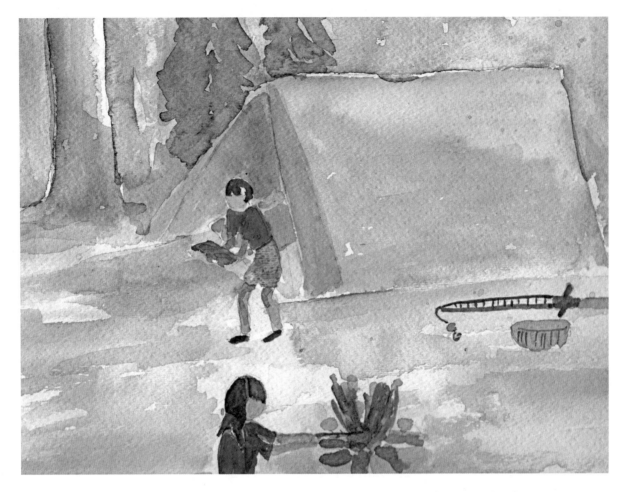

*Did you go camping with your own family or with friends? If you went fishing, describe what it felt like to catch a fish. Did you roast marshmallows? Did you like them burnt or golden brown? What did they taste like? Where did you go hiking? Where did you sleep? Which wild animals did you see? What other activities did you do while camping? What songs did you sing?*

# I Remember

## BUILDING SANDCASTLES

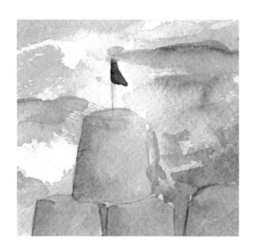

Building castles in the sand

Sets my spirit free.

Sand coats my knees, my legs, my hands.

Almost every part of me!

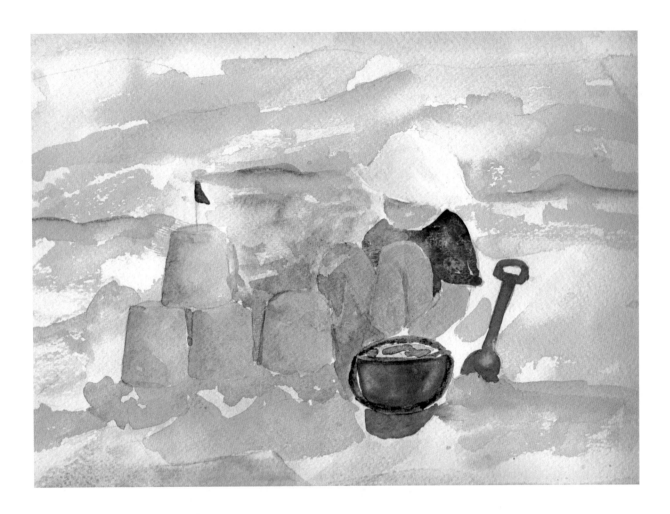

*Have you ever been to the ocean? Who did you go with? What did the waves sound like? What sounds did the sea gulls make? Did you swim in the ocean? Was the water cold? What kind of seashells did you see? What kind of structures did you build? What dried between your toes and on your feet and legs? Tell about what you ate for lunch. What did you enjoy most about your time spent at the ocean?*

# I Remember
# AUTUMN

# I Remember
## RAKING LEAVES

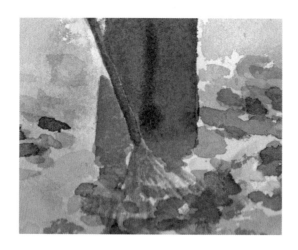

Mr. Wind, please stay away.

We are raking leaves today!

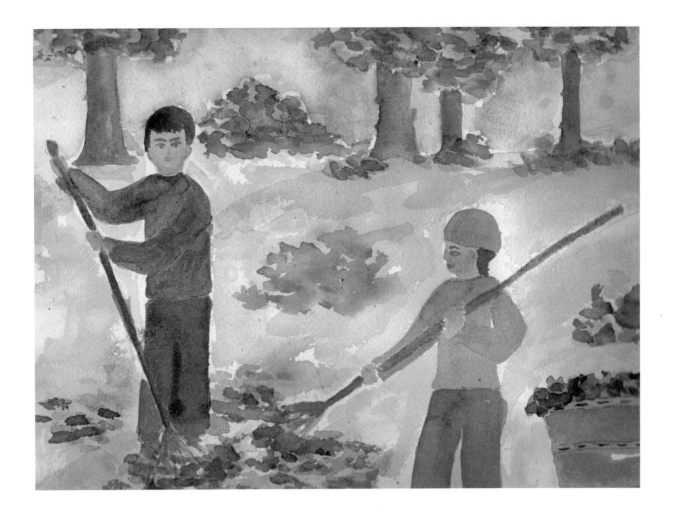

*What was the most fun about raking leaves? Did you rake with someone else? Who was it? How did you play in the leaves? How did the fall leaves smell? When the leaves were all raked, did you bag them or burn them?*

# I Remember
## GOING ON HAYRIDES

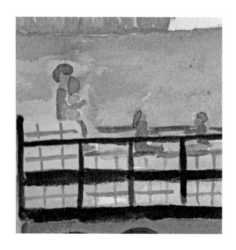

High atop the wagon

On bales of itchy hay,

With a signal to the driver,

Our ride gets underway.

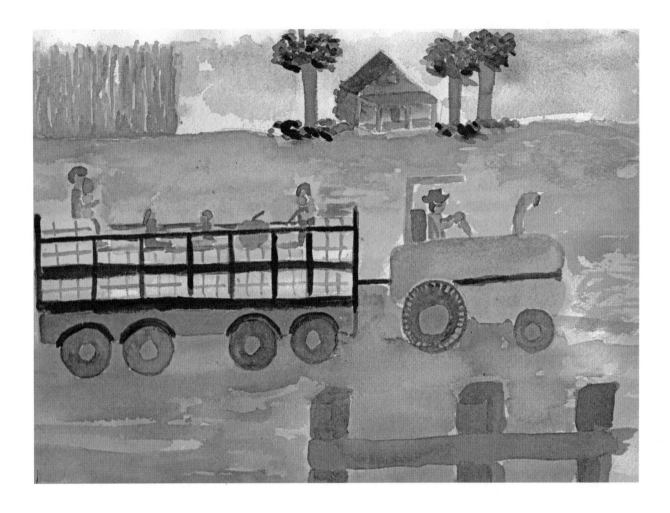

*Have you ever gone on a hayride? Who did you go with? Who, or what, pulled the wagon? What did the hay feel and smell like? What songs did you sing? Did you have a bonfire afterward? What did you roast?*

# I Remember
## HARVEST TIME

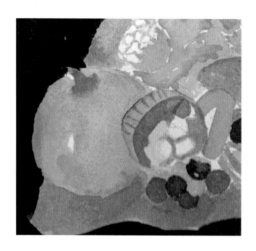

We are thankful for the harvest,

Rows of corn, and fields of wheat.

Just as the farmers promised,

We've delicious food to eat!

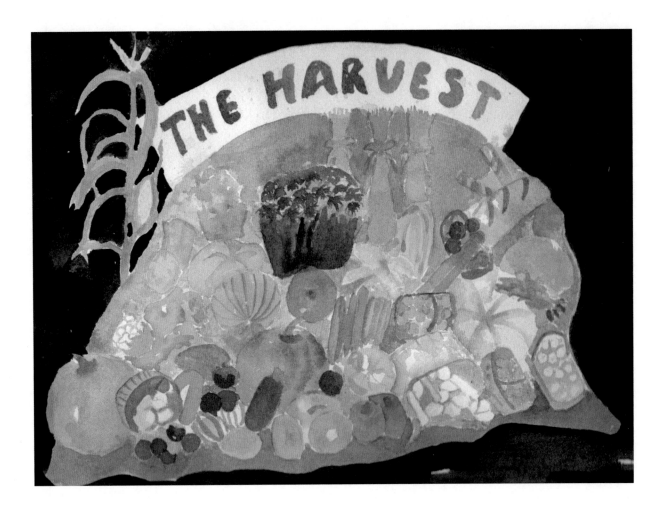

Have you ever seen crops harvested? Name some of the fruits and vegetables. If you helped with harvesting, what was your job? Describe how you did it. What are your favorite foods? What does it mean to be thankful?

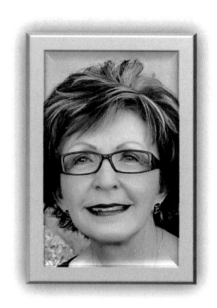

Brenda Poulos is the best-selling author of *Runaways: The Long Journey Home* and *The Choice: Will's Last Testament.*

Brenda divides her time between writing, volunteering, and remodeling projects. She is an avid reader and movie buff, who lives in Mesa, Arizona with her husband John and their two aging pets, Baxter and Brinkley. They have four adult children and seven grandchildren.

A former elementary school teacher and counselor, Brenda maintains two websites, www.spiritualsnippets.com and www.brendapoulos.org. You can also connect with her on Facebook, Goodreads, and Twitter @Mtnst14Brenda.

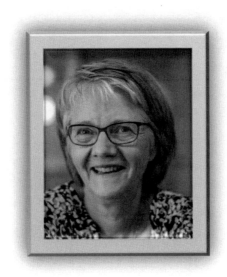

Janis Cox has been blogging since 2008. She is the author/illustrator of two award-winning children's books, *The Kingdom of Thrim* and *Tadeo Turtle*.

She is a weekly contributor to Hope Stream Radio, an Internet radio station. She and her husband live in Haliburton, Ontario but spend winter months in Arizona.

In addition to a career as a homemaker and elementary school teacher, Janis was a partner in a Canadian small business with her husband. They have 3 married children and 7 grandchildren.

Janis can be reached on her website, www.janiscox.com and on Twitter @authorjaniscox.

# Activities for People With Alzheimer's

1. Recite nursery rhymes
2. Listen to music
3. Toss a ball
4. Blow bubbles
5. Sort and fold laundry
6. Color pictures
7. Clip coupons
8. Garden
9. Sort things by shape/color
10. Rake leaves
11. Look at family photos
12. String beads
13. Sweep a patio, porch, or sidewalk
14. Do puzzles
15. Play board games
16. Work with clay
17. Paint pictures; fingerpaint5. 5.
18. Fill a birdfeeder
19. Make a scrapbook
20. Wash windows
21. Sort coins into a container
22. Roll yarn into a ball
23. Dance to favorite music
24. Play a musical instrument
25. Read picture books
26. Add your own ideas

# Games/Activities for use People with Alzheimer's

www.alz.org

www.alzfdn.org

www.best-alzheimers-products.com/games-for-people-with-alzheimers.html

www.keepingbusy.com

https://minddesigngames.com

# Current Research/Statistics

www.alz.org

www.alzheimers.net/resources-alzheimers-statistics

www.theguardian.com

www.terrypierce.com

**Note:** There are literally hundreds of Internet articles available under the headings of Dementia and/or Alzheimer's. We encourage you to do additional reading on your own.

Made in the USA
Las Vegas, NV
21 April 2024

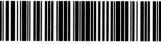